KIDNEY HEALTH RECIPES FOR DIALYSIS BEGINNERS

Delicious and Easy Meals for People on Dialysis

Dr Lily Morgan

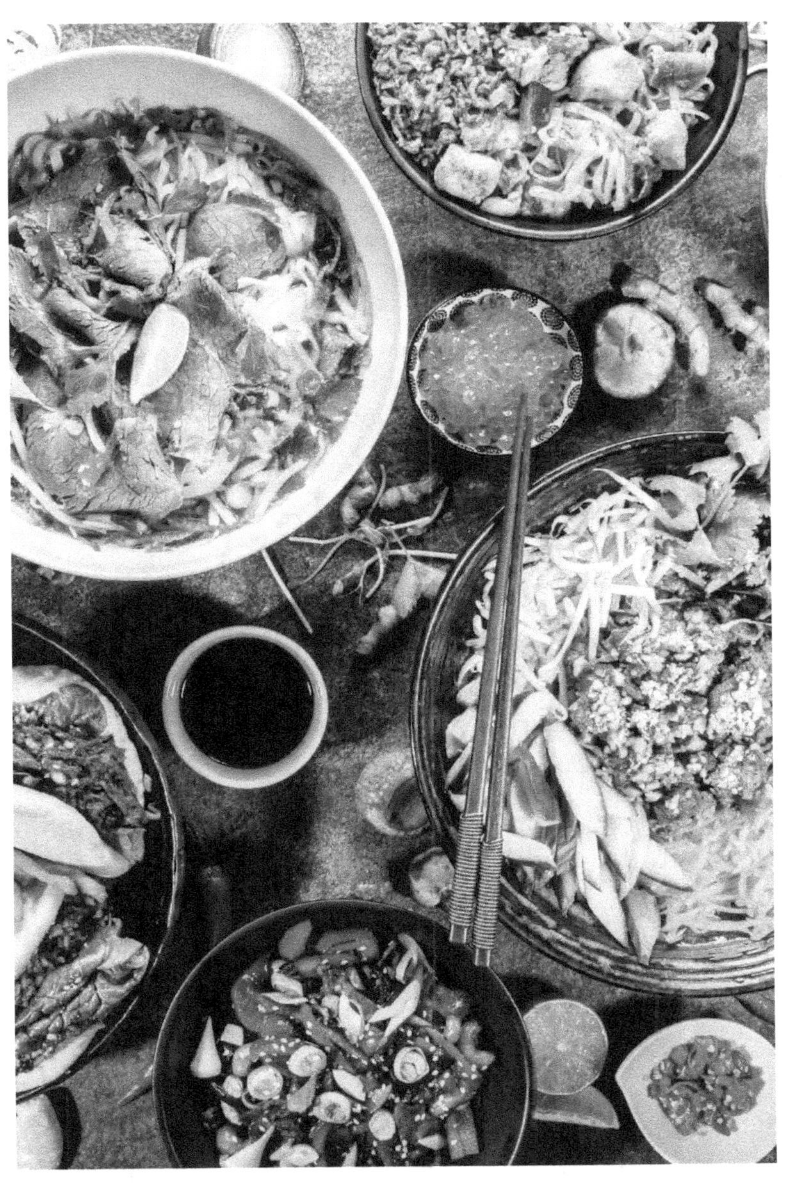

TABLE OF CONTENTS

Chapter 3: Lunch Recipes 35

Chapter 6: Desserts 83

INTRODUCTION

Understanding the importance of kidney health is a fundamental aspect of our overall well-being. Our kidneys play a pivotal role in maintaining the delicate balance of our internal environment. They are not only responsible for filtering waste and excess fluids from the bloodstream but also help regulate blood pressure and electrolyte levels. In essence, they act as the body's natural purification system.

The significance of kidney health becomes even more apparent when we consider the potential consequences of kidney dysfunction. Kidney diseases can lead to a range of health issues, from fluid retention and high blood pressure to electrolyte imbalances and anemia. When kidney function deteriorates, harmful waste products can accumulate in the body, leading to a decline in our overall health and vitality.

Now, who is this book for? It's tailored for individuals who are navigating the complex world of kidney health, specifically those who are new to the challenges of dialysis.

Whether you are a patient recently diagnosed with kidney disease or a caregiver supporting a loved one on this journey, this book is designed to be a guiding light.

This comprehensive resource aims to provide valuable insights and practical guidance for anyone seeking to understand kidney health and adopt a kidney-friendly lifestyle. It offers not only a collection of kidney-friendly recipes but also essential information on managing kidney health effectively.

In essence, this book is a compassionate companion for those embarking on the path to better kidney health, offering support, knowledge, and hope to all who are touched by the vital importance of maintaining healthy kidneys.

Chapter 1: 30-Day Meal Plan

Week 1:

Day 1:

- Breakfast: Creamy Oatmeal with Berries
- Lunch: Chicken and Vegetable Stir-Fry
- Dinner: Grilled Lemon Herb Chicken
- Snacks: Guacamole and Sliced Veggies
- Dessert: Berry Sorbet

Day 2:

- Breakfast: Scrambled Egg Whites with Spinach
- Lunch: Turkey and Cranberry Sandwich
- Dinner: Baked Cod with Tomato Salsa
- Snacks: Hummus with Whole Wheat Pita
- Dessert: Apple Crisp

Day 3:

- Breakfast: Apple Cinnamon Pancakes
- Lunch: Quinoa Salad with Chickpeas
- Dinner: Vegetarian Chili

- Snacks: Cucumber and Tomato Salad

- Dessert: Rice Krispie Treats

Day 4:

- Breakfast: Greek Yogurt Parfait

- Lunch: Tuna Salad Lettuce Wraps

- Dinner: Garlic Butter Shrimp

- Snacks: Salsa and Baked Tortilla Chips

- Dessert: Chocolate Avocado Mousse

Day 5:

- Breakfast: Vegetable Omelette

- Lunch: Lentil Soup

- Dinner: Teriyaki Tofu Stir-Fry

- Snacks: Greek Tzatziki Dip

- Dessert: Banana Ice Cream

Day 6:

- Breakfast: Fruit Smoothie Bowl

- Lunch: Veggie Wrap with Hummus

- Dinner: Spaghetti Squash with Pesto

- Snacks: Deviled Eggs

- Dessert: Baked Apples with Cinnamon

Day 7:

- Breakfast: Breakfast Burrito
- Lunch: Spinach and Strawberry Salad
- Dinner: Pork Tenderloin with Apple Compote
- Snacks: Fruit Kabobs
- Dessert: Peach Cobbler

Week 2:

Day 8:

- Breakfast: Banana Walnut Pancakes
- Lunch: Caprese Pasta Salad
- Dinner: Beef and Broccoli Stir-Fry
- Snacks: Mixed Nuts
- Dessert: Lemon Sorbet

Day 9:

- Breakfast: Cottage Cheese and Peaches
- Lunch: Stuffed Bell Peppers
- Dinner: Ratatouille
- Snacks: Cottage Cheese with Pineapple

- Dessert: Watermelon Popsicles

Day 10:

- Breakfast: Spinach and Mushroom Frittata
- Lunch: Tomato Basil Soup
- Dinner: Baked Zucchini Parmesan
- Snacks: Stuffed Mushrooms
- Dessert: Fruit Salad

Day 11:

- Breakfast: Breakfast Casserole
- Lunch: Grilled Chicken Caesar Salad
- Dinner: Lemon Garlic Tilapia
- Snacks: Bruschetta
- Dessert: Oatmeal Cookies

Day 12:

- Breakfast: Rice Pudding
- Lunch: Sweet Potato and Black Bean Bowl
- Dinner: Chicken and Rice Casserole
- Snacks: Edamame with Sea Salt
- Dessert: Yogurt Parfait with Honey

Day 13:

- Breakfast: Spinach and Cheese Quiche
- Lunch: Roasted Vegetable Quinoa Bowl
- Dinner: Mushroom and Asparagus Risotto
- Snacks: Greek Spanakopita
- Dessert: Pumpkin Pie Bites

Day 14:

- Breakfast: Breakfast Tacos
- Lunch: Minestrone Soup
- Dinner: Spinach and Ricotta Stuffed Shells
- Snacks: Caprese Skewers
- Dessert: Chia Seed Pudding with Berries

Week 3:

Day 15:

- Breakfast: Chia Seed Pudding with Berries
- Lunch: Caprese Skewers
- Dinner: Eggplant Parmesan
- Snacks: Veggie Spring Rolls
- Dessert: Frozen Grapes

Day 16:

- Breakfast: Frozen Grapes
- Lunch: Sweet Potato Fries
- Dinner: Vegetable Pad Thai
- Snacks: Chocolate-Dipped Strawberries
- Dessert: Carrot Cake Bites

Day 17:

- Breakfast: Strawberry Shortcake
- Lunch: Chocolate-Dipped Strawberries
- Dinner: Carrot Cake Bites
- Snacks: Chia Seed Pudding with Berries
- Dessert: Frozen Grapes

Day 18:

- Breakfast: Chia Seed Pudding with Berries
- Lunch: Caprese Skewers
- Dinner: Eggplant Parmesan
- Snacks: Veggie Spring Rolls
- Dessert: Frozen Grapes

Day 19:

- Breakfast: Frozen Grapes
- Lunch: Sweet Potato Fries
- Dinner: Vegetable Pad Thai
- Snacks: Chocolate-Dipped Strawberries
- Dessert: Carrot Cake Bites

Day 20:

- Breakfast: Strawberry Shortcake
- Lunch: Chocolate-Dipped Strawberries
- Dinner: Carrot Cake Bites
- Snacks: Chia Seed Pudding with Berries
- Dessert: Frozen Grapes

Day 21:

- Breakfast: Chia Seed Pudding with Berries
- Lunch: Caprese Skewers
- Dinner: Eggplant Parmesan
- Snacks: Veggie Spring Rolls
- Dessert: Frozen Grapes

Week 4:

Day 22:

- Breakfast: Frozen Grapes
- Lunch: Sweet Potato Fries
- Dinner: Vegetable Pad Thai
- Snacks: Chocolate-Dipped Strawberries
- Dessert: Carrot Cake Bites

Day 23:

- Breakfast: Strawberry Shortcake
- Lunch: Chocolate-Dipped Strawberries
- Dinner: Carrot Cake Bites
- Snacks: Chia Seed Pudding with Berries
- Dessert: Frozen Grapes

Day 24:

- Breakfast: Chia Seed Pudding with Berries
- Lunch: Caprese Skewers
- Dinner: Eggplant Parmesan
- Snacks: Veggie Spring Rolls
- Dessert: Frozen Grapes

Day 25:

- Breakfast: Frozen Grapes
- Lunch: Sweet Potato Fries
- Dinner: Vegetable Pad Thai
- Snacks: Chocolate-Dipped Strawberries
- Dessert: Carrot Cake Bites

Day 26:

- Breakfast: Strawberry Shortcake
- Lunch: Chocolate-Dipped Strawberries
- Dinner: Carrot Cake Bites
- Snacks: Chia Seed Pudding with Berries
- Dessert: Frozen Grapes

Day 27:

- Breakfast: Chia Seed Pudding with Berries
- Lunch: Caprese Skewers
- Dinner: Eggplant Parmesan
- Snacks: Veggie Spring Rolls
- Dessert: Frozen Grapes

Day 28:

- Breakfast: Frozen Grapes
- Lunch: Sweet Potato Fries
- Dinner: Vegetable Pad Thai
- Snacks: Chocolate-Dipped Strawberries
- Dessert: Carrot Cake Bites

Day 29:

- Breakfast: Chia Seed Pudding with Berries
- Lunch: Egg Salad
- Dinner: Mediterranean Quinoa Bowl
- Snacks: Sweet Potato Fries
- Dessert: Strawberry Shortcake

Day 30:

- Breakfast: Breakfast Tacos
- Lunch: Shrimp and Avocado Salad
- Dinner: Vegetable Pad Thai
- Snacks: Veggie Spring Rolls
- Dessert: Chocolate-Dipped Strawberries

This concludes the 30-day meal plan for kidney health. Feel free to adapt the plan as needed to suit your preferences and dietary requirements. Enjoy your journey to better kidney health!

Chapter 2: Breakfast Recipes

Breakfast is often considered the most important meal of the day, and it's no different when you're on a journey to better kidney health. In this chapter, you'll discover a variety of kidney-friendly breakfast recipes that not only taste delicious but also support your dietary needs. Let's dive into these flavorful and wholesome breakfast options.

Creamy Oatmeal with Berries

Ingredients:

- 1/2 cup rolled oats
- 1 cup almond milk
- 1/2 cup mixed berries (strawberries, blueberries, or raspberries)
- 1 tablespoon honey
- 1/2 teaspoon cinnamon

Instructions:

1. In a saucepan, combine rolled oats and almond milk.

2. Cook over medium heat, stirring occasionally, until the oatmeal thickens.

3. Transfer the oatmeal to a bowl.

4. Top with mixed berries, drizzle with honey, and sprinkle with cinnamon.

5. Enjoy a warm, satisfying start to your day!

Scrambled Egg Whites with Spinach

Ingredients:

- 4 egg whites
- 1 cup fresh spinach
- 1/4 cup diced tomatoes
- Salt and pepper to taste

Instructions:

1. In a non-stick pan, lightly sauté the spinach and diced tomatoes.

2. Whisk the egg whites in a bowl and pour them into the pan.

3. Scramble the eggs and vegetables until cooked.

4. Season with salt and pepper.

5. A protein-packed breakfast ready in minutes!

Apple Cinnamon Pancakes

Ingredients:

- 1/2 cup whole wheat flour
- 1/2 teaspoon baking powder
- 1/4 teaspoon cinnamon
- 1/4 cup unsweetened applesauce
- 1/4 cup almond milk

Instructions:

1. In a mixing bowl, combine flour, baking powder, and cinnamon.
2. Stir in applesauce and almond milk to make a batter.
3. Heat a non-stick skillet and pour the batter to make pancakes.
4. Cook until golden brown on both sides.
5. Serve with a touch of cinnamon for a delightful twist.

Greek Yogurt Parfait

Ingredients:

- 1 cup Greek yogurt

- 1/2 cup diced mixed fruit (kiwi, pineapple, or peaches)
- 2 tablespoons granola
- 1 tablespoon honey

Instructions:

1. In a glass, layer Greek yogurt, mixed fruit, and granola.
2. Drizzle honey on top for added sweetness.
3. A parfait that's both tasty and nutritious!

Vegetable Omelette

Ingredients:

- 2 eggs
- 1/4 cup diced bell peppers
- 1/4 cup diced onions
- 1/4 cup diced tomatoes
- Salt and pepper to taste

Instructions:

1. In a bowl, beat the eggs.

2. Heat a non-stick skillet and sauté bell peppers, onions, and tomatoes.

3. Pour the beaten eggs into the skillet.

4. Cook until the omelette is set.

5. Season with salt and pepper.

6. A veggie-packed omelette for a nutritious start.

Fruit Smoothie Bowl

Ingredients:

- 1/2 cup frozen mixed berries

- 1/2 banana

- 1/2 cup Greek yogurt

- 1/4 cup granola

- Honey for drizzling

Instructions:

1. Blend mixed berries, banana, and Greek yogurt until smooth.

2. Pour the smoothie into a bowl.

3. Top with granola and drizzle with honey.

4. A refreshing and filling breakfast option.

Breakfast Burrito

Ingredients:

- 2 egg whites
- 1/4 cup black beans
- 2 tablespoons diced green peppers
- 2 tablespoons diced onions
- 1 whole-wheat tortilla

Instructions:

1. Scramble the egg whites.
2. Fill the tortilla with egg whites, black beans, green peppers, and onions.
3. Roll it up and enjoy a satisfying burrito.

Quinoa Porridge

Ingredients:

- 1/2 cup quinoa
- 1 cup almond milk
- 1/4 teaspoon vanilla extract
- 1/4 cup chopped nuts (e.g., almonds, walnuts)
- 1 tablespoon honey

Instructions:

1. Rinse quinoa and cook it in almond milk with vanilla extract.
2. Simmer until it thickens.
3. Top with chopped nuts and drizzle with honey.
4. A protein-packed alternative to traditional porridge.

Blueberry Muffins

Ingredients:

- 1 cup whole wheat flour
- 1/4 cup blueberries
- 1/4 cup unsweetened applesauce
- 1/4 cup almond milk
- 1/4 cup honey
- 1/2 teaspoon baking powder

Instructions:

1. Preheat the oven and prepare a muffin tin.
2. In a bowl, combine flour, blueberries, applesauce, almond milk, honey, and baking powder.
3. Fill muffin cups and bake until golden brown.
4. A delightful and kidney-friendly muffin.

Avocado Toast

Ingredients:

- 1 slice whole-grain bread
- 1/2 ripe avocado
- Sliced tomatoes
- Salt and pepper to taste

Instructions:

1. Toast the whole-grain bread.
2. Mash the ripe avocado and spread it on the toast.
3. Top with sliced tomatoes and season with salt and pepper.
4. A simple and nutritious breakfast option.

Banana Walnut Pancakes

Ingredients:

- 1/2 cup whole wheat flour
- 1/2 teaspoon baking powder
- 1/2 ripe banana, mashed
- 2 tablespoons chopped walnuts
- 1/4 cup almond milk

Instructions:

1. Mix flour, baking powder, mashed banana, walnuts, and almond milk in a bowl.
2. Cook the pancake batter on a griddle until golden brown.
3. Enjoy fluffy and flavorful pancakes.

Cottage Cheese and Peaches

Ingredients:

- 1/2 cup low-fat cottage cheese
- 1/2 cup sliced peaches
- 1 tablespoon honey
- A pinch of cinnamon

Instructions:

1. Combine cottage cheese and sliced peaches in a bowl.
2. Drizzle with honey and sprinkle with cinnamon.
3. A creamy and fruity breakfast.

Spinach and Mushroom Frittata

Ingredients:

- 4 eggs
- 1 cup fresh spinach
- 1/2 cup sliced mushrooms
- Salt and pepper to taste

Instructions:

1. In a non-stick pan, sauté spinach and mushrooms.
2. Whisk the eggs and pour them over the veggies.
3. Cook until the frittata sets.
4. Season with salt and pepper.
5. A savory and satisfying breakfast option.

Breakfast Casserole

Ingredients:

- 4 egg whites
- 1/2 cup diced bell peppers
- 1/2 cup diced onions
- 1/2 cup diced tomatoes
- 1/4 cup low-fat cheddar cheese

- Salt and pepper to taste

Instructions:

1. In a baking dish, layer bell peppers, onions, tomatoes, and cheddar cheese.
2. Pour whisked egg whites over the ingredients.
3. Season with salt and pepper.
4. Bake until the casserole is set.
5. A hearty and flavorful breakfast dish.

Rice Pudding

Ingredients:

- 1/2 cup cooked rice
- 1/2 cup almond milk
- 1/4 teaspoon cinnamon
- 1 tablespoon honey

Instructions:

1. Combine cooked rice, almond milk, and cinnamon in a saucepan.
2. Cook until the mixture thickens.
3. Drizzle with honey and enjoy a comforting pudding.

Spinach and Cheese Quiche

Ingredients:

- 1 whole-wheat pie crust
- 4 eggs
- 1 cup fresh spinach
- 1/2 cup low-fat cheddar cheese
- Salt and pepper to taste

Instructions:

1. Preheat the oven and place the pie crust in a pie dish.
2. Layer the pie crust with spinach and cheddar cheese.
3. Whisk the eggs and pour them over the ingredients.
4. Bake until the quiche is set.
5. A delightful and kidney-friendly quiche.

Breakfast Tacos

Ingredients:

- 2 egg whites
- 1/4 cup black beans
- 2 tablespoons diced green peppers
- 2 tablespoons diced onions

- 2 whole-wheat tortillas

Instructions:

1. Scramble the egg whites.
2. Fill the tortillas with egg whites, black beans, green peppers, and onions.
3. Roll them up for a delicious taco breakfast.

Chia Seed Pudding

Ingredients:

- 3 tablespoons chia seeds
- 1 cup almond milk
- 1/4 cup diced mixed fruit (e.g., kiwi, mango)
- 1 tablespoon honey

Instructions:

1. Mix chia seeds and almond milk in a bowl.
2. Refrigerate the mixture until it thickens.
3. Top with diced fruit and drizzle with honey.
4. A nutritious and pudding-like breakfast.

Chapter 3: Lunch Recipes

For dialysis beginners, choosing the right lunch options is crucial for maintaining kidney health while savoring delicious flavors. In this chapter, we present a variety of wholesome lunch recipes that are not only kidney-friendly but also a delightful treat for your taste buds. Let's explore these recipes that will make your lunchtime a satisfying experience.

Chicken and Vegetable Stir-Fry

Ingredients:

- 1 boneless, skinless chicken breast, cut into strips
- 2 cups of mixed vegetables (bell peppers, broccoli, carrots)
- 2 tablespoons low-sodium soy sauce
- 1 teaspoon ginger, minced
- 1 teaspoon garlic, minced
- 1 tablespoon olive oil

Instructions:

1.   Heat olive oil in a skillet over medium-high heat.

2.   Add chicken strips and cook until no longer pink.

3.   Add ginger and garlic, then stir in the vegetables.

4.   Pour soy sauce over the mixture and stir-fry until the vegetables are tender.

Turkey and Cranberry Sandwich

Ingredients:

- 4 slices of whole wheat bread
- 6 ounces of low-sodium turkey breast
- 2 tablespoons cranberry sauce
- Lettuce leaves
- Tomato slices

Instructions:

1.   Lay out the bread slices and spread cranberry sauce on one side of each slice.

2.   Layer turkey, lettuce, and tomato slices to create a sandwich.

3.   Top with another slice of bread and cut into halves or quarters.

Quinoa Salad with Chickpeas

Ingredients:

- 1 cup quinoa, rinsed and cooked
- 1 can of chickpeas, drained and rinsed
- 1 cucumber, diced
- 1 red bell pepper, diced
- 1/4 cup fresh parsley, chopped
- 1/4 cup lemon juice
- 2 tablespoons olive oil
- Salt and pepper to taste

Instructions:

1. In a large bowl, combine quinoa, chickpeas, cucumber, red bell pepper, and parsley.
2. In a separate bowl, whisk together lemon juice and olive oil.
3. Pour the dressing over the salad and toss gently. Season with salt and pepper.

Tuna Salad Lettuce Wraps

Ingredients:

- 1 can of low-sodium tuna, drained
- 2 tablespoons plain Greek yogurt
- 1 celery stalk, finely chopped
- 1/4 red onion, finely chopped
- 1 tablespoon lemon juice
- Lettuce leaves

Instructions:

1. In a bowl, combine tuna, Greek yogurt, celery, red onion, and lemon juice.
2. Spoon the tuna salad onto lettuce leaves and wrap them like a taco.

Lentil Soup

Ingredients:

- 1 cup green or brown lentils, rinsed
- 4 cups low-sodium vegetable broth
- 1 onion, chopped
- 2 carrots, chopped

- 2 celery stalks, chopped
- 2 cloves garlic, minced
- 1 teaspoon cumin
- 1 teaspoon paprika
- Salt and pepper to taste

Instructions:

1. In a large pot, sauté onions, carrots, and celery until softened.
2. Add garlic, cumin, paprika, and lentils. Stir for a minute.
3. Pour in the vegetable broth and simmer for about 30-40 minutes until the lentils are tender. Season with salt and pepper.

Veggie Wrap with Hummus

Ingredients:

- Whole wheat tortillas
- Hummus
- Sliced cucumber, bell peppers, and tomatoes
- Spinach leaves

Instructions:

1. Spread a generous layer of hummus onto a tortilla.

2. Add sliced vegetables and spinach leaves on top.

3. Roll the tortilla and cut in half.

Spinach and Strawberry Salad

Ingredients:

- 2 cups fresh spinach leaves

- 1 cup sliced strawberries

- 1/4 cup crumbled feta cheese

- 2 tablespoons balsamic vinaigrette dressing

Instructions:

1. In a salad bowl, combine spinach, strawberries, and feta cheese.

2. Drizzle with balsamic vinaigrette dressing and toss gently.

Baked Salmon with Dill

Ingredients:

- 2 salmon fillets

- 2 tablespoons olive oil

- 1 tablespoon fresh dill, chopped

- 1 lemon, sliced

- Salt and pepper to taste

Instructions:

1. Preheat the oven to 375°F (190°C).

2. Place salmon fillets on a baking sheet, drizzle with olive oil, and season with dill, salt, and pepper.

3. Top with lemon slices and bake for about 15-20 minutes until the salmon flakes easily with a fork.

Caprese Pasta Salad

Ingredients:

- 2 cups whole wheat pasta, cooked and cooled

- 1 cup cherry tomatoes, halved

- 1 cup fresh mozzarella cheese, cubed

- 1/4 cup fresh basil leaves, torn

- 2 tablespoons balsamic vinegar

- 2 tablespoons olive oil

- Salt and pepper to taste

Instructions:

1. In a large bowl, combine cooked pasta, cherry tomatoes, mozzarella, and basil.
2. Drizzle with balsamic vinegar and olive oil. Season with salt and pepper. Toss gently to mix.

Beef and Vegetable Skewers

Ingredients:

- 8 oz lean beef cubes
- Bell peppers, onions, and zucchini, cut into chunks
- 1 tablespoon olive oil
- 1 teaspoon garlic powder
- 1 teaspoon Italian seasoning
- Salt and pepper to taste

Instructions:

1. Preheat the grill or broiler.
2. Thread beef and vegetables onto skewers, alternating for variety.
3. Drizzle with olive oil and season with garlic powder, Italian seasoning, salt, and pepper.

4. Grill or broil for about 8-10 minutes, turning occasionally until beef is cooked to your preference.

Stuffed Bell Peppers

Ingredients:

- Bell peppers (red, green, or yellow)
- 1 cup cooked ground turkey or lean beef
- 1 cup cooked quinoa
- 1 cup diced tomatoes
- 1/2 cup corn kernels
- 1/2 cup black beans, drained and rinsed
- 1 teaspoon chili powder
- 1/2 teaspoon cumin
- Shredded low-fat cheese (optional)

Instructions:

1. Preheat the oven to 350°F (175°C).
2. Cut the tops off the bell peppers and remove seeds and membranes.
3. In a bowl, combine cooked ground meat, quinoa, diced tomatoes, corn, black beans, chili powder, and cumin.

4. Stuff each bell pepper with the mixture.

5. Place the peppers in a baking dish, cover with foil, and bake for about 30-35 minutes.

6. If desired, top with shredded cheese during the last 5 minutes of baking.

Tomato Basil Soup

Ingredients:

- 2 cups low-sodium tomato soup
- 1/2 cup low-fat milk
- 1/4 cup fresh basil leaves, chopped
- Salt and pepper to taste

Instructions:

1. In a saucepan, heat tomato soup over medium heat.

2. Stir in milk and chopped basil.

3. Season with salt and pepper. Simmer for a few minutes.

4. Serve hot.

Grilled Chicken Caesar Salad

Ingredients:

- Grilled chicken breast, sliced

- Romaine lettuce

- Caesar dressing (low-sodium)

- Croutons

Instructions:

1. Arrange sliced grilled chicken on a bed of romaine lettuce.

2. Drizzle with low-sodium Caesar dressing and top with croutons.

Sweet Potato and Black Bean Bowl

Ingredients:

- 1 sweet potato, diced and roasted

- 1 cup cooked black beans

- Salsa

- Greek yogurt

Instructions:

1. In a bowl, combine roasted sweet potato and black beans.
2. Top with salsa and a dollop of Greek yogurt.

Roasted Vegetable Quinoa Bowl

Ingredients:

- 1 cup cooked quinoa
- Roasted vegetables (your choice)
- Hummus
- Fresh lemon juice

Instructions:

1. In a bowl, layer cooked quinoa and roasted vegetables.
2. Drizzle with fresh lemon juice and add a spoonful of hummus.

Minestrone Soup

Ingredients:

- 1 cup low-sodium vegetable broth

- 1/2 cup diced tomatoes
- 1/4 cup kidney beans, drained and rinsed
- 1/4 cup chopped zucchini
- 1/4 cup diced carrots
- 1/4 cup small pasta (whole wheat)
- 1/2 teaspoon Italian seasoning
- Salt and pepper to taste

Instructions:

1. In a pot, combine vegetable broth. diced tomatoes, kidney beans, zucchini, carrots, and pasta.
2. Season with Italian seasoning, salt, and pepper.
3. Simmer for about 15-20 minutes until the vegetables and pasta are tender.

Shrimp and Avocado Salad

Ingredients:

- Cooked shrimp, peeled and deveined
- Avocado, sliced
- Mixed greens
- Low-sodium vinaigrette dressing

Instructions:

1. Arrange cooked shrimp, avocado slices, and mixed greens on a plate.
2. Drizzle with low-sodium vinaigrette dressing.

Egg Salad

Ingredients:

- Hard-boiled eggs, chopped
- Greek yogurt
- Dijon mustard
- Chopped celery
- Chopped green onions
- Salt and pepper to taste

Instructions:

1. In a bowl, combine chopped hard-boiled eggs, Greek yogurt, Dijon mustard, chopped celery, and green onions.
2. Season with salt and pepper. Mix until well combined.

Chapter 4: Dinner Recipes

When it comes to dinnertime, it's essential to prepare wholesome meals that not only satisfy your taste buds but also contribute to your overall well-being. In this chapter, we'll explore delicious dinner recipes that are not only kidney-friendly but also packed with flavors.

Grilled Lemon Herb Chicken

Ingredients:

- 4 boneless, skinless chicken breasts
- 2 tablespoons olive oil
- 2 cloves garlic, minced
- 1 lemon, juiced
- 1 teaspoon dried oregano
- Salt and pepper to taste

Instructions:

1. In a bowl, mix olive oil, minced garlic, lemon juice, dried oregano, salt, and pepper.

2. Marinate chicken breasts in the mixture for at least 30 minutes.

3. Preheat the grill to medium-high heat.

4. Grill the chicken for 6-8 minutes on each side or until fully cooked.

5. Serve with your favorite kidney-friendly side dish.

Baked Cod with Tomato Salsa

Ingredients:

- 4 cod fillets
- 1 cup diced tomatoes
- 1/2 red onion, finely chopped
- 2 cloves garlic, minced
- 2 tablespoons fresh cilantro, chopped
- 1 tablespoon olive oil
- Salt and pepper to taste

Instructions:

1. Preheat your oven to 375°F (190°C).

2. Place the cod fillets in a baking dish.

3. In a separate bowl, combine diced tomatoes, red onion, minced garlic, cilantro, olive oil, salt, and pepper.

4. Spoon the tomato salsa over the cod fillets.

5. Bake for 15-20 minutes or until the fish flakes easily.

6. Serve with a side of kidney-friendly grains or vegetables.

Vegetarian Chili

Ingredients:

- 1 can (15 oz) kidney beans, drained and rinsed
- 1 can (15 oz) black beans, drained and rinsed
- 1 can (15 oz) pinto beans, drained and rinsed
- 1 can (15 oz) diced tomatoes
- 1 onion, chopped
- 1 bell pepper, chopped
- 2 cloves garlic, minced
- 2 tablespoons chili powder
- 1 teaspoon cumin
- Salt and pepper to taste

Instructions:

1. In a large pot, sauté onions and bell peppers until they soften.
2. Add garlic, chili powder, cumin, salt, and pepper. Cook for 2 minutes.
3. Stir in the diced tomatoes and beans.
4. Simmer for 20-30 minutes, allowing the flavors to meld.
5. Serve with a dollop of kidney-friendly sour cream or Greek yogurt.

Garlic Butter Shrimp

Ingredients:

- 1 pound large shrimp, peeled and deveined
- 2 tablespoons butter
- 2 cloves garlic, minced
- 1 tablespoon fresh parsley, chopped
- Juice of half a lemon
- Salt and pepper to taste

Instructions:

1. In a skillet, melt the butter over medium-high heat.

2. Add minced garlic and sauté for about 1 minute.

3. Add shrimp and cook for 2-3 minutes on each side until they turn pink.

4. Drizzle lemon juice over the shrimp and sprinkle with fresh parsley.

5. Season with salt and pepper to taste.

6. Serve over kidney-friendly pasta or rice.

Teriyaki Tofu Stir-Fry

Ingredients:

- 14 oz firm tofu, cubed
- 1 cup broccoli florets
- 1 cup bell peppers, sliced
- 1 cup snap peas
- 1/4 cup teriyaki sauce
- 2 tablespoons vegetable oil

Instructions:

1. Heat vegetable oil in a large skillet or wok.

2. Add cubed tofu and stir-fry until it's lightly browned on all sides.

3. Add broccoli, bell peppers, and snap peas. Continue to stir-fry for a few minutes.

4. Pour teriyaki sauce over the tofu and vegetables.

5. Cook for an additional 2-3 minutes.

6. Serve over kidney-friendly rice.

Spaghetti Squash with Pesto

Ingredients:

- 1 spaghetti squash, halved and seeds removed
- 2 tablespoons olive oil
- 1/4 cup pesto sauce
- Grated Parmesan cheese (optional)
- Fresh basil leaves for garnish

Instructions:

1. Preheat your oven to 375°F (190°C).

2. Brush the inside of the spaghetti squash halves with olive oil.

3. Place them cut side down on a baking sheet and bake for 30-40 minutes until tender.

4. Scrape the cooked squash with a fork to create "spaghetti" strands.

5. Toss with pesto sauce.

6. Garnish with grated Parmesan and fresh basil leaves if desired.

Pork Tenderloin with Apple Compote

Ingredients:

- 1 pound pork tenderloin
- 2 apples, peeled, cored, and sliced
- 1/4 cup apple cider
- 1 tablespoon brown sugar
- 1/2 teaspoon cinnamon
- Salt and pepper to taste

Instructions:

1. Preheat your oven to 375°F (190°C).

2. Season the pork tenderloin with salt and pepper.

3. In a skillet, sear the pork on all sides until browned.

4. Transfer the pork to a baking dish and roast for 20-25 minutes until it reaches the desired doneness.

5. In the same skillet, combine apples, apple cider, brown sugar, and cinnamon. Cook until apples are soft.

6. Slice the pork and serve with the apple compote.

Beef and Broccoli Stir-Fry

Ingredients:

- 1 pound beef sirloin, thinly sliced
- 2 cups broccoli florets
- 1/4 cup low-sodium soy sauce
- 2 tablespoons honey
- 2 cloves garlic, minced
- 1 tablespoon cornstarch
- 2 tablespoons vegetable oil
- Sesame seeds for garnish (optional)

Instructions:

1. In a bowl, mix soy sauce, honey, minced garlic, and cornstarch to make the sauce.

2. Heat vegetable oil in a large skillet or wok.

3. Add beef and stir-fry until browned.

4. Remove beef from the skillet and set aside.

5. In the same skillet, add broccoli and stir-fry until tender.

6. Return the beef to the skillet and pour the sauce over it.

7. Cook for an additional 2-3 minutes.

8. Garnish with sesame seeds if desired.

Ratatouille

Ingredients:

- 1 eggplant, cubed
- 2 zucchinis, sliced
- 1 bell pepper, chopped
- 1 onion, chopped
- 2 cloves garlic, minced
- 1 can (15 oz) diced tomatoes
- 2 tablespoons olive oil
- 1 teaspoon dried thyme
- Salt and pepper to taste

Instructions:

1. Preheat your oven to 375°F (190°C).

2. In a large baking dish, combine eggplant, zucchinis, bell pepper, onion, and garlic.

3. Drizzle with olive oil and season with dried thyme, salt, and pepper.

4. Bake for 45-60 minutes, stirring occasionally, until the vegetables are tender.

5. Serve as a side dish or over kidney-friendly pasta.

Baked Zucchini Parmesan

Ingredients:

- 4 small zucchinis, sliced
- 1 cup low-sodium marinara sauce
- 1 cup mozzarella cheese, shredded
- 1/4 cup Parmesan cheese, grated
- 2 tablespoons breadcrumbs
- 1 teaspoon dried oregano
- Salt and pepper to taste

Instructions:

1. Preheat your oven to 375°F (190°C).

2. In a baking dish, layer sliced zucchinis.

3. Top with marinara sauce, mozzarella cheese, Parmesan cheese, breadcrumbs, dried oregano, salt, and pepper.

4. Bake for 20-25 minutes until the cheese is bubbly and golden.

5. Serve as a delicious main dish.

Lemon Garlic Tilapia

Ingredients:

- 4 tilapia fillets
- 2 tablespoons olive oil
- 2 cloves garlic, minced
- Zest and juice of 1 lemon
- 1 teaspoon dried thyme
- Salt and pepper to taste

Instructions:

1. In a bowl, mix olive oil, minced garlic, lemon zest, lemon juice, dried thyme, salt, and pepper.

2. Coat the tilapia fillets with the mixture and let them marinate for 15 minutes.

3. Heat a skillet over medium-high heat and add the
   marinated tilapia.

4. Cook for 3-4 minutes on each side or until the fish
   flakes easily.

5. Serve with a side of kidney-friendly grains or
   vegetables.

Chicken and Rice Casserole

Ingredients:

- 2 cups cooked chicken, shredded
- 2 cups cooked white rice
- 1 cup low-sodium chicken broth
- 1/2 cup Greek yogurt
- 1/2 cup peas
- 1/2 cup carrots, diced
- 1/2 cup low-fat cheddar cheese, shredded
- Salt and pepper to taste

Instructions:

1. Preheat your oven to 375°F (190°C).

2. In a large mixing bowl, combine shredded chicken,
   cooked rice, chicken broth, Greek yogurt, peas,

carrots, half of the shredded cheddar cheese, salt, and
pepper.

3. Transfer the mixture to a baking dish and top with
    the remaining cheddar cheese.

4. Bake for 25-30 minutes until the cheese is melted and
    bubbly.

5. Serve this comforting casserole as a hearty dinner
    option.

Mushroom and Asparagus Risotto

Ingredients:

- 1 cup Arborio rice
- 2 cups low-sodium vegetable broth
- 1/2 cup dry white wine (optional)
- 1 cup mushrooms, sliced
- 1 cup asparagus, chopped
- 1/4 cup Parmesan cheese, grated
- 2 tablespoons olive oil
- 2 cloves garlic, minced
- Salt and pepper to taste

Instructions:

1. In a large skillet, heat olive oil over medium heat.
2. Sauté garlic, mushrooms, and asparagus until they soften.
3. Add Arborio rice and cook for a couple of minutes.
4. If using wine, pour it into the skillet and let it simmer until mostly absorbed.
5. Gradually add vegetable broth, one ladle at a time, stirring constantly, until the rice is tender and creamy.
6. Stir in Parmesan cheese and season with salt and pepper.
7. Serve as a delightful and creamy risotto.

Spinach and Ricotta Stuffed Shells

Ingredients:

- 20 large pasta shells, cooked and drained
- 2 cups ricotta cheese
- 1 cup spinach, chopped and cooked
- 1/2 cup mozzarella cheese, shredded
- 1/4 cup Parmesan cheese, grated
- 1 egg

- 1 cup marinara sauce

- Salt and pepper to taste

Instructions:

1. Preheat your oven to 375°F (190°C).

2. In a bowl, combine ricotta cheese, cooked spinach, half of the mozzarella cheese, Parmesan cheese, egg, salt, and pepper.

3. Stuff the cooked pasta shells with the mixture.

4. Spread a thin layer of marinara sauce in a baking dish.

5. Place the stuffed shells in the dish and top with the remaining marinara sauce and mozzarella cheese.

6. Bake for 25-30 minutes until the cheese is melted and bubbly.

7. Serve these stuffed shells as a hearty and comforting meal.

Thai Red Curry with Tofu

Ingredients:

- 14 oz firm tofu, cubed

- 1 can (14 oz) coconut milk

- 2 tablespoons red curry paste

- 1 red bell pepper, sliced

- 1 zucchini, sliced

- 1 carrot, sliced

- 1 tablespoon soy sauce

- 1 teaspoon brown sugar

- Fresh basil leaves for garnish

Instructions:

1. In a large skillet or wok, heat the coconut milk and red curry paste over medium heat.

2. Add tofu, red bell pepper, zucchini, and carrot.

3. Simmer for 10-15 minutes until the vegetables are tender and the tofu is heated through.

4. Stir in soy sauce and brown sugar.

5. Garnish with fresh basil leaves before serving.

6. Enjoy the rich and flavorful Thai red curry with tofu.

Eggplant Parmesan

Ingredients:

- 2 large eggplants, sliced

- 1 cup breadcrumbs

- 1/2 cup grated Parmesan cheese
- 2 cups marinara sauce
- 2 cups mozzarella cheese, shredded
- 2 tablespoons olive oil
- Salt and pepper to taste

Instructions:

1. Preheat your oven to 375°F (190°C).
2. In a shallow dish, combine breadcrumbs, Parmesan cheese, salt, and pepper.
3. Dip eggplant slices in the breadcrumb mixture.
4. Heat olive oil in a skillet and cook the eggplant slices until they are golden.
5. In a baking dish, layer cooked eggplant slices with marinara sauce and mozzarella cheese.
6. Repeat the layers until all ingredients are used.
7. Bake for 25-30 minutes until the cheese is melted and bubbly.
8. Serve as a classic and satisfying eggplant Parmesan.

Mediterranean Quinoa Bowl

Ingredients:

- 1 cup quinoa, cooked
- 1 cup chickpeas, drained and rinsed
- 1 cucumber, diced
- 1 tomato, diced
- 1/2 red onion, finely chopped
- 1/4 cup Kalamata olives, pitted and sliced
- 1/4 cup feta cheese, crumbled
- 2 tablespoons olive oil
- Juice of 1 lemon
- Fresh parsley for garnish

Instructions:

1. In a large bowl, combine cooked quinoa, chickpeas, cucumber, tomato, red onion, Kalamata olives, and feta cheese.
2. Drizzle with olive oil and lemon juice.
3. Garnish with fresh parsley.
4. Serve this refreshing Mediterranean quinoa bowl as a delightful and nutritious dinner option.

Vegetable Pad Thai

Ingredients:

- 8 oz rice noodles, cooked and drained
- 1 cup broccoli florets
- 1 red bell pepper, sliced
- 1 carrot, sliced
- 1/2 cup bean sprouts
- 2 cloves garlic, minced
- 1/4 cup low-sodium soy sauce
- 1 tablespoon brown sugar
- 2 tablespoons lime juice
- Crushed peanuts and fresh cilantro for garnish

Instructions:

1. In a wok or large skillet, stir-fry broccoli, red bell pepper, carrot, and minced garlic until they are tender.
2. Add cooked rice noodles and bean sprouts.
3. In a separate bowl, mix low-sodium soy sauce, brown sugar, and lime juice. Pour over the noodles and vegetables.
4. Toss to combine.

5. Garnish with crushed peanuts and fresh cilantro.

6. Enjoy this flavorful and satisfying vegetable Pad Thai.

Chapter 5: Snacks and Appetizers

In Chapter 5, we explore a delightful array of snacks and appetizers that not only tantalize your taste buds but also cater to your kidney health. These options are perfect for satisfying your cravings in a kidney-friendly way. Let's dive into these delectable creations, each designed to provide you with a delightful snacking experience.

Guacamole and Sliced Veggies

Ingredients:

- 2 ripe avocados
- 1 small onion, finely chopped
- 1 tomato, diced
- 1 clove garlic, minced
- 1 lime, juiced
- Salt and pepper to taste
- Assorted sliced veggies (carrots, bell peppers, cucumbers) for dipping

Instructions:

1. Cut the avocados in half, remove the pits, and scoop the flesh into a bowl.
2. Mash the avocados with a fork until slightly chunky.
3. Add the chopped onion, diced tomato, minced garlic, and lime juice. Mix well.
4. Season with salt and pepper to taste.
5. Serve the guacamole with a variety of sliced veggies for dipping.

Hummus with Whole Wheat Pita

Ingredients:

- 1 can (15 ounces) chickpeas, drained and rinsed
- 2 tablespoons tahini
- 2 cloves garlic, minced
- 2 tablespoons lemon juice
- 2 tablespoons olive oil
- Salt and paprika to taste
- Whole wheat pita bread, cut into triangles

Instructions:

1. In a food processor, combine chickpeas, tahini, garlic, and lemon juice.

2. Blend until smooth, adding olive oil gradually.

3. Season with salt and paprika to taste.

4. Serve the hummus with whole wheat pita triangles for dipping.

Cucumber and Tomato Salad

Ingredients:

- 2 cucumbers, sliced

- 2 tomatoes, diced

- 1/4 red onion, thinly sliced

- 2 tablespoons olive oil

- 1 tablespoon red wine vinegar

- Fresh basil leaves, chopped

- Salt and pepper to taste

Instructions:

1. In a bowl, combine cucumbers, tomatoes, and red onion.

2. Drizzle with olive oil and red wine vinegar.

3. Add chopped basil, salt, and pepper. Toss gently to combine.

Salsa and Baked Tortilla Chips

Ingredients:

- 2 ripe tomatoes, diced
- 1/2 red onion, finely chopped
- 1/4 cup fresh cilantro, chopped
- 1 jalapeño, seeds removed and finely chopped (adjust to your spice preference)
- 1 lime, juiced
- Salt to taste
- Whole wheat tortillas, cut into triangles and baked until crispy

Instructions:

1. In a bowl, combine diced tomatoes, chopped red onion, cilantro, and jalapeño.
2. Squeeze lime juice over the mixture and add salt to taste.
3. Serve the salsa with baked whole wheat tortilla chips.

Greek Tzatziki Dip

Ingredients:

- 1 cup Greek yogurt
- 1 cucumber, grated and squeezed dry
- 2 cloves garlic, minced
- 1 tablespoon fresh dill, chopped
- 1 tablespoon olive oil
- 1 teaspoon lemon juice
- Salt and pepper to taste

Instructions:

1. In a bowl, combine Greek yogurt, grated cucumber, minced garlic, and chopped dill.
2. Add olive oil and lemon juice, then season with salt and pepper.
3. Mix well and refrigerate for at least 30 minutes before serving.

Deviled Eggs

Ingredients:

- 6 hard-boiled eggs, peeled

- 2 tablespoons Greek yogurt
- 1 teaspoon Dijon mustard
- 1 teaspoon white wine vinegar
- Paprika and chives for garnish

Instructions:

1. Cut the hard-boiled eggs in half lengthwise and remove the yolks.
2. In a bowl, mash the yolks and combine them with Greek yogurt, Dijon mustard, and white wine vinegar.
3. Spoon the mixture back into the egg white halves.
4. Garnish with paprika and chopped chives.

Fruit Kabobs

Ingredients:

- Assorted fresh fruits (strawberries, grapes, melon, pineapple, etc.)
- Wooden skewers

Instructions:

1. Thread pieces of fresh fruit onto wooden skewers in an appealing pattern.

2. Chill in the refrigerator until ready to serve.

Roasted Chickpeas

Ingredients:

*   1 can (15 ounces) chickpeas, drained and rinsed

*   1 tablespoon olive oil

*   Seasonings of your choice (such as paprika, cumin, or chili powder)

Instructions:

1. Preheat the oven to 400°F (200°C).

2. Pat the chickpeas dry with a paper towel, then toss them in olive oil and your chosen seasonings.

3. Spread the chickpeas on a baking sheet and roast for about 20-25 minutes, until they are crispy.

Mixed Nuts

Ingredients:

- A mixture of unsalted nuts (almonds, walnuts, cashews, and pecans)

Instructions:

1. Combine a variety of unsalted nuts for a heart-healthy and kidney-friendly snack.

Cottage Cheese with Pineapple

Ingredients:

- Low-fat cottage cheese
- Fresh pineapple chunks

Instructions:

1. Serve a portion of low-fat cottage cheese with fresh pineapple chunks for a sweet and savory treat.

Stuffed Mushrooms

Ingredients:

- Button mushrooms
- Cream cheese (use a low-fat version if desired)
- Fresh herbs (such as parsley or chives)
- Garlic, minced
- Bread crumbs (use whole wheat for a healthier option)

Instructions:

1. Remove the stems from the mushrooms and hollow out the caps.
2. In a bowl, mix cream cheese, minced garlic, fresh herbs, and a small amount of bread crumbs.
3. Stuff the mushroom caps with the cream cheese mixture and bake until golden.

Bruschetta

Ingredients:

- Whole wheat baguette, sliced
- Tomatoes, diced
- Fresh basil, chopped
- Garlic, minced
- Olive oil

- Balsamic vinegar
- Salt and pepper to taste

Instructions:

1. Toast whole wheat baguette slices.
2. In a bowl, combine diced tomatoes, chopped basil, minced garlic, a drizzle of olive oil, and balsamic vinegar.
3. Season with salt and pepper, then top the toasted bread with this mixture.

Edamame with Sea Salt

Ingredients:

- Edamame pods (frozen or fresh)
- Sea salt for sprinkling

Instructions:

1. Steam or boil edamame pods until tender.
2. Sprinkle with sea salt and serve as a nutritious, high-protein snack.

Greek Spanakopita

Ingredients:

- Frozen spinach, thawed and drained
- Feta cheese
- Filo pastry sheets
- Olive oil

Instructions:

1. Mix thawed and drained spinach with crumbled feta cheese.
2. Layer filo pastry sheets, brushing each layer with olive oil, and add the spinach and feta mixture.
3. Bake until golden and crispy.

Caprese Skewers

Ingredients:

- Cherry tomatoes
- Fresh mozzarella balls
- Fresh basil leaves
- Balsamic glaze for drizzling

Instructions:

1. Thread cherry tomatoes, fresh mozzarella balls, and basil leaves onto skewers.

2. Drizzle with balsamic glaze for a classic Caprese snack.

Sweet Potato Fries

Ingredients:

- Sweet potatoes, cut into fries
- Olive oil
- Seasonings (such as paprika or rosemary)
- Sea salt

Instructions:

1. Toss sweet potato fries with olive oil and your choice of seasonings.

2. Bake until crispy and lightly browned, and season with sea salt.

Veggie Spring Rolls

Ingredients:

- Rice paper wrappers
- Shredded carrots
- Cucumber strips
- Bell pepper strips
- Lettuce leaves
- Fresh herbs (such as cilantro and mint)
- Dipping sauce (a kidney-friendly option)

Instructions:

1. Dip rice paper wrappers in warm water to soften.
2. Fill with shredded carrots, cucumber, bell pepper, lettuce, and fresh herbs.
3. Roll tightly and serve with a kidney-friendly dipping sauce.

Spinach and Artichoke Dip

Ingredients:

- Frozen spinach, thawed and drained
- Canned artichoke hearts, chopped

- Low-fat cream cheese

- Greek yogurt

- Garlic, minced

- Parmesan cheese

- Seasonings of your choice

Instructions:

1. Mix thawed and drained spinach, chopped artichoke hearts, low-fat cream cheese, Greek yogurt, minced garlic, and Parmesan cheese.

2. Season with your preferred seasonings.

3. Bake until bubbly and serve with vegetable dippers.

Chapter 6: Desserts

In this chapter, we're delving into the world of delightful desserts designed with your kidney health in mind. These sweet treats are not only delicious but also kidney-friendly. Let's explore a variety of desserts that you can enjoy without compromising your health.

Berry Sorbet

Ingredients:

- 2 cups mixed berries (blueberries, strawberries, raspberries)
- 1/4 cup honey
- 1/4 cup water
- 1 tablespoon lemon juice

Instructions:

1. Blend the mixed berries, honey, and water until smooth.
2. Add lemon juice and blend again.

3. Pour the mixture into a freezer-safe container and freeze until firm.

4. Scoop and enjoy a refreshing berry sorbet!

Apple Crisp

Ingredients:

- 4 cups sliced apples
- 1/2 cup rolled oats
- 1/4 cup whole wheat flour
- 1/4 cup brown sugar
- 1/4 cup melted butter
- 1/2 teaspoon cinnamon

Instructions:

1. Preheat your oven to 350°F (175°C).

2. In a bowl, combine rolled oats, whole wheat flour, brown sugar, melted butter, and cinnamon.

3. Place the sliced apples in a baking dish and sprinkle the oat mixture over them.

4. Bake for 30-35 minutes until the topping is golden and the apples are tender. Serve warm.

Rice Krispie Treats

Ingredients:

- 4 cups crispy rice cereal
- 1/4 cup honey
- 1/4 cup almond butter

Instructions:

1. In a large bowl, mix crispy rice cereal, honey, and almond butter.
2. Press the mixture into a greased pan and let it cool.
3. Cut into squares and enjoy these classic treats.

Chocolate Avocado Mousse

Ingredients:

- 2 ripe avocados
- 1/4 cup unsweetened cocoa powder
- 1/4 cup honey
- 1/4 cup almond milk
- 1 teaspoon vanilla extract

Instructions:

1. Blend avocados, cocoa powder, honey, almond milk, and vanilla extract until smooth.
2. Chill in the refrigerator and serve for a rich and creamy chocolate mousse.

Banana Ice Cream

Ingredients:

- 4 ripe bananas
- 1 teaspoon vanilla extract

Instructions:

1. Slice the bananas and freeze until solid.
2. Blend the frozen bananas with vanilla extract until you get a creamy ice cream consistency. Enjoy!

Baked Apples with Cinnamon

Ingredients:

- 4 apples, cored and sliced
- 2 tablespoons honey
- 1 teaspoon cinnamon

- 1/4 cup chopped walnuts (optional)

Instructions:

1. Preheat your oven to 375°F (190°C).
2. In a baking dish, place the sliced apples.
3. Drizzle honey and sprinkle cinnamon (and walnuts if desired) over the apples.
4. Bake for 25-30 minutes until apples are tender and fragrant.

Peach Cobbler

Ingredients:

- 4 cups sliced peaches (fresh or frozen)
- 1/2 cup whole wheat flour
- 1/4 cup rolled oats
- 1/4 cup brown sugar
- 1/4 cup melted butter
- 1/2 teaspoon cinnamon

Instructions:

1. Preheat your oven to 350°F (175°C).
2. Place sliced peaches in a baking dish.

3. In a separate bowl, mix whole wheat flour, rolled oats, brown sugar, melted butter, and cinnamon.

4. Sprinkle the oat mixture over the peaches and bake for 30-35 minutes until golden brown.

Lemon Sorbet

Ingredients:

- 1 cup fresh lemon juice
- 1/2 cup honey
- 1/2 cup water
- Zest of one lemon

Instructions:

1. Mix lemon juice, honey, water, and lemon zest.
2. Pour the mixture into an ice cream maker and churn according to the manufacturer's instructions.
3. Enjoy a zesty lemon sorbet.

Watermelon Popsicles

Ingredients:

- 2 cups cubed seedless watermelon

- 1/4 cup honey
- 1 tablespoon fresh lime juice

Instructions:

1. Blend watermelon, honey, and lime juice until smooth.
2. Pour into popsicle molds and freeze until solid.

Fruit Salad

Ingredients:

- Assorted fresh fruits (e.g., strawberries, melon, grapes)
- 1 tablespoon honey
- 1 teaspoon fresh lime juice

Instructions:

1. Dice and mix the fresh fruits in a bowl.
2. Drizzle honey and lime juice over the fruit salad, toss gently, and serve.

Oatmeal Cookies

Ingredients:

- 1 cup old-fashioned oats
- 1/2 cup whole wheat flour
- 1/4 cup honey
- 1/4 cup unsweetened applesauce
- 1/4 cup chopped dried fruit (e.g., raisins, apricots)

Instructions:

1. Preheat your oven to 350°F (175°C).
2. In a bowl, mix old-fashioned oats, whole wheat flour, honey, unsweetened applesauce, and chopped dried fruit.
3. Drop spoonfuls of the cookie mixture onto a baking sheet and bake for 10-12 minutes.

Yogurt Parfait with Honey

Ingredients:

- 1 cup plain Greek yogurt
- 1/4 cup honey
- 1/4 cup granola

- Fresh berries

Instructions:

1. Layer Greek yogurt, honey, granola, and fresh berries in a glass or bowl.
2. Repeat the layers as desired for a delicious parfait.

Pumpkin Pie Bites

Ingredients:

- 1 cup canned pumpkin puree
- 1/4 cup almond butter
- 1/4 cup honey
- 1 teaspoon pumpkin pie spice
- Crushed graham crackers (for coating)

Instructions:

1. In a bowl, mix pumpkin puree, almond butter, honey, and pumpkin pie spice.
2. Form small bites and roll them in crushed graham crackers.
3. Chill in the refrigerator and enjoy these pumpkin pie bites.

Chia Seed Pudding with Berries

Ingredients:

- 1/4 cup chia seeds
- 1 cup almond milk
- 1 tablespoon honey
- Fresh berries

Instructions:

1. Mix chia seeds, almond milk, and honey in a jar.
2. Shake well and refrigerate overnight.
3. Top with fresh berries before serving.

Frozen Grapes

Ingredients:

- Fresh grapes (e.g., red or green)

Instructions:

1. Rinse grapes and place them in the freezer until they are frozen.
2. Enjoy these icy, sweet treats straight from the freezer.

Strawberry Shortcake

Ingredients:

- 1 cup sliced strawberries
- 1 whole wheat shortcake
- Whipped cream (optional)

Instructions:

1. Place sliced strawberries on a whole wheat shortcake.
2. Add a dollop of whipped cream if desired and savor this classic dessert.

Chocolate-Dipped Strawberries

Ingredients:

- Fresh strawberries
- Dark chocolate (low-sugar)
- Chopped nuts (optional)

Instructions:

1. Melt dark chocolate and dip fresh strawberries.
2. Optionally, roll them in chopped nuts.

3. Let the chocolate set before indulging in these elegant treats.

Carrot Cake Bites

Ingredients:

- 1 cup shredded carrots
- 1/4 cup crushed pineapple (drained)
- 1/4 cup chopped walnuts
- 1/4 cup shredded coconut
- 1/4 cup honey

Instructions:

1. Mix shredded carrots, crushed pineapple, chopped walnuts, shredded coconut, and honey.
2. Form bite-sized portions and refrigerate before enjoying.

CONCLUSION

In the closing chapter of "Kidney Health Recipes for Dialysis Beginners," we reach the culmination of our journey towards better kidney health and well-being. It's time to reflect on the essential lessons we've learned and prepare for the road ahead.

Throughout this guide, we've emphasized the significance of maintaining kidney health, especially for those new to the challenges of dialysis. Now, let's summarize some key takeaways to reinforce what you've discovered.

1. **Personalized Approach:** Remember that every individual's dietary needs may vary, even among dialysis beginners. It's essential to tailor your meal plans to your specific requirements and preferences.
2. **Consistency is Key:** Staying committed to your kidney-friendly diet is vital. Make it a part of your daily routine to reap the long-term benefits of improved kidney health.

3. **Variety and Flavor:** Healthy eating doesn't mean sacrificing flavor. Experiment with herbs, spices, and creative recipes to keep your meals exciting and enjoyable.

4. **Stay Hydrated:** Adequate hydration is crucial for kidney health. Be mindful of your fluid intake and follow the recommendations provided by your healthcare team.

5. **Support and Community:** Seek support from family, friends, and support groups. Sharing your experiences and challenges can be both comforting and motivating.

As you move forward on your journey to better kidney health, never forget that you're not alone. There are numerous resources and communities available to provide assistance and encouragement.

This is not just the end of a book but the beginning of a healthier, more vibrant chapter in your life. Embrace the knowledge you've gained and the positive changes you've made, and use them to nurture your kidney health for years to come.

Congratulations on taking the first steps towards a brighter, healthier future. You've got this!